COPING WITH DEMENTIA

The Complete Guide to Managing Your Symptoms for Dementia Patients, Loved Ones, and Caregivers

Dr. C. ROLAND

Table of Contents

CHAPTER ONE
Introduction

Dementia is a widespread and complex neurological disorder that has a substantial impact on the lives of persons affected and those in their immediate surroundings. This introduction provides an entry point into the tremendous complexities of dementia, laying the groundwork for comprehending the condition and its repercussions. Our investigation includes not only the clinical but also the emotional and practical aspects of living with dementia.

Defined Dementia

Dementia is a wide word that refers to a group of symptoms caused by a deterioration in cognitive function that interferes with daily life. Memory loss, decreased communication, diminished intellectual ability, and difficulties executing ordinary tasks are some of the symptoms. While dementia is more common in older people, it is critical to dispel the myth that it is an inevitable component of the aging process.

This tutorial aims to demystify dementia's varied nature by diving into its numerous forms. From the most frequent variety, Alzheimer's disease, to vascular dementia, Lewy body dementia, and frontotemporal dementia, each subtype has its own set of obstacles. Individuals, caregivers, and loved ones can modify their approach to better meet the specific requirements of those living with dementia by understanding these distinctions.

Understanding the Implications

Aside from the medical complexities, dementia has a significant influence on individuals, families, and communities. It tests the very foundations of relationships and routines, necessitating modifications and adaptation. Individuals diagnosed with dementia may experience feelings of frustration and loss as their cognitive functions deteriorate. Meanwhile, family members and loved ones frequently find themselves negotiating a difficult emotional landscape, combining the need to provide care with the person with dementia's dignity and autonomy.

Why Is This Guide Important?

This guide is more than just a collection of facts; it is a tribute to the value of knowledge and compassion in the face of dementia. Our goal as we delve into the complexities of this disorder is to provide readers with a full grasp of dementia—its origins, progression, and the numerous ways it presents.

We recognize the emotional burden that comes with a dementia diagnosis, as well as the problems that caregivers encounter. As a result, our handbook is intended to be a useful resource for patients, their loved ones, and those who provide care. We hope to promote a sense of support and community by providing practical insights, coping skills, and a holistic perspective.

Join us on this trip as we explore the multifaceted world of dementia, hoping to inspire understanding and empathy as much as to inform. Together, we can pave the way for more awareness, compassionate care, and improved quality of life for individuals affected by dementia.

❖ The Importance of Symptom Management

Understanding and efficiently managing dementia symptoms are critical components in improving the quality of life for those diagnosed with the condition, as well as their loved ones and caregivers. This section examines the relevance of proactive symptom management and its far-reaching impact on the well-being of dementia patients.

❖ Dementia Symptom Dynamics

Dementia symptoms can appear in a variety of ways, impacting cognitive abilities, emotional well-being, and daily activities. Memory loss, forgetfulness, difficulty speaking, mood swings, and difficulties performing simple chores are all common symptoms. If left untreated, these symptoms can lead to increased frustration, anxiety, and a loss of independence in people with dementia.

❖ Patients' Quality of Life

Proactive symptom management directly contributes to those living with dementia retaining a higher quality of life. It entails adapting care techniques to individual symptoms, providing therapies that boost cognitive function, and creating a secure environment. Individuals with dementia may benefit from improved cognitive functioning, improved emotional well-being, and increased engagement in daily activities as a result of this process.

❖ Relationship Preservation for Loved Ones

Understanding and managing dementia symptoms is critical for loved ones in maintaining relationships and emotional ties. Effective communication strategies, empathy, and patience become critical in managing the changes that occur as dementia progresses. Loved ones can contribute to a more stable and supportive atmosphere by addressing symptoms early on, creating pleasant interactions and moments of shared joy.

❖ Reducing the Burden of Caregiving

Caregivers, who play an important part in the daily care of people with dementia, can confront substantial problems. The value of symptom management extends to reducing caregiver burden by providing them with the tools and knowledge they need to deliver good care. Understanding the intricacies of each symptom, implementing practical strategies for assistance, and seeking help when necessary are all part of it. Caregivers can maintain their own well-being and provide better care to their loved ones by proactively managing symptoms.

❖ A Holistic Approach to Happiness

Beyond specific symptoms, a holistic approach to well-being management is critical. This includes taking into account the physical, emotional, and social aspects of dementia patients. A holistic approach to symptom treatment must include activities that generate joy, promote physical health, and create social connections.

Educating and Empowering the Target Audience

This handbook acknowledges that effective symptom management requires a team effort from patients, loved ones, and caregivers. It is designed to provide each group with knowledge and tactics that are specific to their jobs. Patients learn about self-care and adaptation, loved ones learn how to provide meaningful support, and caregivers get practical advice on negotiating the intricacies of caregiving.

Dementia: An Overview

Dementia is a complex and frequently difficult disorder that affects cognitive skills, such as memory, reasoning, and daily activities. For novices, learning the basics of dementia entails investigating its various varieties, comprehending potential causes and risk factors, and recognizing common symptoms and the evolution of the disorder.

Dementia Types

Dementia is a broad term that refers to a variety of cognitive problems. Each type has distinct traits and may progress in different ways. Here are some examples of common dementias:

1. **Alzheimer's disease**, the most common form of dementia, is defined by the buildup of aberrant protein deposits in the brain, resulting in the slow degeneration of brain cells.

2. Vascular dementia: is caused by decreased blood flow to the brain, which is mainly caused by strokes or other vascular disorders. It is the most frequent type of dementia.

3. Lewy Body Dementia: This form is characterized by abnormal protein deposits in the brain known as Lewy bodies. It is frequently characterized by cognitive oscillations, visual hallucinations, and movement symptoms resembling Parkinson's disease.

4. Frontotemporal Dementia: This type of dementia typically affects the frontal and temporal lobes of the brain, resulting in personality, behavior, and language abnormalities.

Understanding the precise form of dementia is critical for adapting treatment and assistance to match the individual and family needs.

Factors of Risk and Causes

The causes of dementia vary, and numerous factors frequently contribute to its development. Some of the most important causes and risk factors are as follows:

1. Age: The risk of dementia increases with age, with persons over 65 accounting for the vast majority of cases.

2. Genetics: Certain genetic variables may predispose persons to dementia, yet this is not the only factor.

3. Brain Injury: Head traumas, especially those that cause brain damage, can raise the risk of dementia.

4. Cardiovascular Health: Heart and blood vessel conditions such as hypertension and diabetes can contribute to the development of vascular dementia.

Understanding these aspects aids in detecting potential risks and, where possible, implementing preventive measures.

Typical Symptoms and Progression

The symptoms of dementia might vary based on the type and stage of the disorder. Typical symptoms include:

1. Forgetfulness, particularly of recent occurrences, is a defining sign.

2. Cognitive decline is characterized by difficulties in reasoning, problem solving, and decision making.

3. Difficulties finding the correct words or expressing thoughts coherently are common communication challenges.

4. Mood swings, impatience, and apathy are common behavioral changes.

5. Impaired Motor Skills: As dementia progresses, people may struggle with coordination and movement.

Dementia progresses gradually in most cases, and the rate varies from person to person. Early detection and intervention can have a substantial impact on the condition's progress and improve the quality of life for patients and their families.

Understanding dementia entails accepting its various manifestations, identifying potential causes, and being acquainted with the prevalent symptoms. This fundamental information serves as the foundation for providing appropriate dementia support and care.

CHAPTER TWO
Dementia Diagnosis and Treatment

Understanding dementia diagnosis and treatment options is critical for both those experiencing symptoms and their caretakers. This section explains the early detection and diagnosis process, medical approaches to dementia, and non-pharmacological therapies in layman's terms.

Diagnosis and detection at an early stage

1. Recognizing and admitting Symptoms: Recognizing and admitting symptoms is the first step in diagnosing dementia. Memory loss, confusion, behavioral problems, and trouble with regular activities are all possible.

2. Consultation with Healthcare Professionals: When symptoms are noted, people or their families often seek consultation with healthcare professionals such as primary care physicians or neurologists.

3. Medical History and Physical Exam: Healthcare practitioners collect a complete medical history, perform a physical exam, and question about the development and course of symptoms. They may also administer cognitive tests to examine memory and thinking ability.

4. Cognitive Testing: Cognitive tests, such as the Mini-Mental State Examination (MMSE) or the Montreal Cognitive Assessment (MoCA), aid in the assessment and diagnosis of various cognitive functions.

5. Imaging techniques, such as CT scans or MRI, can be used to detect structural abnormalities in the brain. This helps to eliminate other probable sources of symptoms.

6. Blood testing can help uncover disorders that may be contributing to cognitive loss, such as vitamin shortages or thyroid issues.

Early detection enables timely intervention, allowing individuals and their families to prepare for the future and adopt appropriate care methods.

Medical Treatments for Dementia

1. Drugs: A number of drugs are approved to treat Alzheimer's disease and other kinds of dementia. These drugs may aid in the improvement of cognitive function, mood, or the

postponement of symptom development.

2. Cholinesterase inhibitors, such as donepezil, rivastigmine, and galantamine, are often used to improve communication between nerve cells.

3. Memantine is another medicine that controls glutamate activity in the brain, with the goal of slowing cognitive decline.

4. Medications for Specific Symptoms: Medications for specific symptoms, such as antipsychotics for behavioral problems or antidepressants for mood-related difficulties, may be recommended.

It's crucial to remember that pharmaceutical effects vary, and not all people with dementia will benefit from pharmacological therapies.

Non-pharmacological Treatments

1. Cognitive Stimulation: Mentally stimulating activities such as puzzles, games, and social interactions can aid in cognitive function maintenance.

2. Regular physical activity has been linked to better cognitive performance and overall well-being.

3. Occupational Therapy: Occupational therapists can help people adapt to daily chores, promote independence, and improve their quality of life.

4. Speech and Language Therapy: Speech therapists can help people who are having difficulty communicating by teaching them ways to improve their verbal expression and comprehension.

5. assistance Groups and Counseling: Individuals with dementia and their caregivers require emotional and psychological assistance. Joining support groups or getting counseling can provide helpful advice and a sense of connection.

Taking Care of the Patient

Understanding how to create a supportive atmosphere, apply appropriate communication tactics, and set daily living activities and routines is critical for novices navigating the obstacles of caring for someone with dementia. This section offers practical tips for caregivers, whether family members or professionals, on how to improve the well-being of people with dementia.

Creating a Friendly Environment

1. First and foremost, ensure that the living space is safe and free of risks. Remove tripping risks, secure sharp objects, and, if necessary, add railings.

2. Maintain a familiar and consistent setting to prevent misunderstanding. Keep personal possessions accessible and minimize changes in furniture arrangement.

3. Adequate Lighting: Maintain well-lit facilities, especially in commonly utilized areas. Proper lighting can help decrease confusion and improve sight.

4. Create quiet and tranquil locations where people can withdraw if they are feeling overwhelmed. Soft colors, comfortable furniture, and familiar items can all help to create a relaxing environment.

5. Memory Aids: To help with orientation and recall, use memory aids such as labels, signs, or visual cues. Labeling drawers and doors can help people find things on their own.

Strategies for Effective Communication

1. Simplify Language: Use simple and straightforward language. Divide instructions or information into smaller, more comprehensible chunks.

2. Maintain Eye Contact: Make and keep eye contact during interactions. Nonverbal clues can help people with dementia communicate better.

3. Patience and Calmness: Be patient and keep your cool. Avoid rushing or displaying frustration, since this can add to the

caregiver's and the individual's stress.

4. Use Visual and Tactile Cues: To reinforce communication, use visual aids, gestures, and touch. Nonverbal cues can be more useful than verbal clues in some situations.

5. Encourage Expression: Encourage free communication by encouraging others to express themselves. Validate their emotions and provide reassurance.

Routines and activities of daily living

1. Create Consistent Routines: Make daily tasks into a routine. Predictability can give comfort and alleviate worry.

2. Break down daily chores into smaller, more doable steps. This

method can make activities more manageable and less intimidating.

3. Encourage Independence: Encourage independence by incorporating the individual to the best of their abilities in daily duties. This could entail getting dressed, grooming, or setting the table.

4. Provide Options: Provide options whenever feasible to empower the individual. Simple decisions, such as deciding between two outfits, might help you feel more in control.

5. Be adaptable: Adaptability is essential. Adapt activities and routines to the preferences and skills of the individual. Flexibility enables a more responsive and supportive approach to caregiving.

In conclusion, caring for someone with dementia entails creating a safe atmosphere, using effective communication tactics, and developing daily routines that add to a sense of familiarity and security. Individuals with dementia can experience enhanced well-being by adopting these concepts into caregiving, and caregivers can negotiate their roles with greater confidence and empathy.

Help for Family Members

For new caregivers navigating the challenges of dementia care, it is critical to understand the emotional and psychological impact on family and friends, develop strategies to balance caregiver obligations, and appreciate the need of obtaining external help. This section offers practical tips and ideas to assist loved ones in dealing with the complications of caregiving.

Family and Friends' Emotional and Psychological Impact

Caring for a dementia patient can elicit a wide range of feelings, from love and compassion to anger and despair. The first step toward providing appropriate support is to understand the emotional and psychological impact:

1. Grief and Loss: Seeing a deterioration in cognitive ability might result in sentiments of grief and loss. It's critical to identify these feelings and give yourself time to absorb them.

2. Stress and Anxiety: The obligations of caregiving, together with observing the hardships faced by the person with dementia, can result in increased stress and anxiety. Self-care becomes critical.

3. Caregivers frequently experience guilt, believing they could do more or questioning their capacity to offer proper care. This can lead to burnout by highlighting the importance of self-compassion.

4. Changes in Role: The dynamic between the caregiver and the person suffering from dementia may vary, affecting relationships and roles. Adapting to these developments necessitates open communication and flexibility.

5. Positive Moments: Despite the difficulties, caring can provide opportunities for joy and connection. Recognizing and cherishing these happy times might help with emotional resiliency.

Caregiver Responsibilities Must Be Balanced

1. Set realistic expectations: Recognize that caring for someone with dementia is a difficult responsibility. It is critical to set reasonable expectations and accept constraints.

2. Delegate Tasks: It is OK to seek assistance and delegate tasks. Family and friends may be willing to share responsibilities, easing the load on the primary caretaker.

3. Establish Regular Breaks: Regular breaks are critical for avoiding burnout. Caregivers require time for themselves, whether it be a quick stroll, time for a hobby, or a social outing.

4. Prioritize Self-Care: Self-care is a necessity, not a luxury. Take care of your physical and emotional well-being by obtaining adequate sleep, eating a good food, and engaging in enjoyable hobbies.

5. Professional Help: Hire professional caregivers or use respite care services to provide brief reprieve and support.

Seeking Outside Help: Support Groups, Counseling, etc.

1. Support Groups: Participating in a caregiver support group helps individuals to share their experiences, acquire insights, and receive emotional support from others facing similar issues.

2. Counseling: Professional counseling can offer caregivers with a safe place to vent their thoughts, discover coping skills, and receive stress management advice.

3. Look for educational materials and resources about dementia and caregiving. Understanding the disease and the available resources

can help caregivers feel more empowered.

4. Respite Care: Use respite care services to offer caregivers a break while ensuring that the person with dementia is cared for by skilled specialists.

5. Legal and Financial Counsel: Seek legal and financial counsel to handle any planning problems. Understanding your alternatives and planning for the future can help reduce the burden of caregiving.

CHAPTER THREE
Holistic Well-Being Approaches

1. Encourage frequent physical activity, even if it's as simple as a gentle walk or seated exercises. Physical well-being benefits general health and can improve mood.

2. Nutrition: Eat a well-balanced, nutritious diet. A well-nourished body promotes cognitive function and supplies the energy required for daily tasks.

3. Sleep hygiene entails developing a consistent sleep habit. Sleep is essential for cognitive performance and emotional well-being.

4. Emotional well-being is addressed by engaging in activities that bring joy and relaxation. Listening to music, enjoying

nature, or indulging in creative activities are all examples of this.

5. Spiritual and Cultural Engagement: Maintain involvement in spiritual or cultural practices, if applicable. These activities can create a sense of belonging and purpose.

Participating in Meaningful Activities

1. Identify Interests: Recognize and continue things that have previously been pleasurable. Hobbies, crafts, and other pastimes can be modified to accommodate existing skills.

2. Activities should be modified based on current cognitive and physical capacities. Simplify activities to keep them enjoyable and attainable.

3. Create a schedule that incorporates familiar and pleasurable activities to structure the day. A sense of security is enhanced by predictability and consistency.

4. Sensory Stimulation: Experiment with activities that stimulate the senses of touch, smell, sight, and hearing. Sensory experiences can elicit memories and improve overall well-being.

5. Involve individuals in meaningful duties such as preparing the table, folding laundry, or gardening. These activities help to create a sense of accomplishment.

Increasing Social Connections

1. Family and Friends: Maintain contact with family and friends. Emotional support and a sense of

belonging are provided by meaningful ties with loved ones.

2. Support Groups: Participating in support groups for people with dementia and their caregivers gives a forum for sharing experiences and receiving mutual support.

3. Participate in community activities or programs designed specifically for people with dementia. This encourages social engagement and a sense of belonging.

4. Volunteer Opportunities: If possible, participate in volunteer activities. Giving back to the community gives you a sense of purpose and success.

5. Interaction with pets can provide companionship as well as emotional support. Animals have

been demonstrated to alleviate stress and promote well-being.

In essence, preserving quality of life for people with dementia entails taking a holistic approach to well-being, engaging in meaningful activities, and fostering social connections. Caregivers and loved ones can contribute to a pleasant and enriching life experience for persons navigating the dementia path by concentrating on these factors.

Considerations for Legal and Financial Considerations

Understanding legal and financial factors is critical for beginners managing the challenges connected with dementia in order to plan for the future, handle anticipated challenges, and obtain necessary assistance. This section includes practical information to assist individuals and families in navigating this portion of the dementia journey.

Making Future Plans

1. Advance Care Planning: Use advance care planning to describe medical care choices, including decisions on life-sustaining therapies. This could include making a living will or naming a healthcare proxy.

2. Consider creating a power of attorney for both healthcare and financial affairs. This legal instrument appoints someone to make decisions on the individual's behalf when they are no longer able to do so.

3. Will and Estate Planning: Consult with a legal practitioner to draft or update a will and to plan a comprehensive estate. This

ensures that assets are dispersed in accordance with the intentions of the individual.

4. Guardianship: When a person is no longer capable of making decisions and has not chosen a power of attorney, families may need to consider guardianship proceedings. This legal procedure appoints a guardian to make decisions on the person with dementia's behalf.

5. Long-Term Care Planning: Research long-term care choices, such as the need for assisted living or nursing facility care. Plan for the fees and look into insurance or government help programs.

Legal and financial difficulties

1. Capacity and Consent: As dementia progresses, the individual's decision-making

capacity may deteriorate. This might cause issues with permission for medical procedures, financial transactions, and legal contracts.

2. Individuals suffering from dementia may be exposed to financial exploitation. Set up precautions such as account monitoring and joint accounts with a trustworthy family member.

3. Medicaid Planning: If you anticipate needing long-term care, look into Medicaid planning alternatives. Medicaid is a federal program that assists qualified persons in covering the costs of medical and long-term care.

4. Financial Management: Managing finances might become difficult as cognitive capacities deteriorate. Consider enlisting the assistance of a trusted family

member or financial professional to help you with bill payments, budgeting, and financial issues.

5. Legal Protections: Be aware that there are legal safeguards against discrimination based on cognitive impairment. These safeguards can include employment, housing, and access to services.

Assistance and Resources

1. Seek counsel from legal practitioners who specialize in elder law or estate planning. They can advise you on legal paperwork, your rights, and your responsibilities.

2. Consult with a financial counselor to plan for the financial implications of dementia care. They can offer advice on financial strategies, retirement planning, and long-term care insurance.

3. Investigate government programs such as Social Security, Medicare, and Medicaid. Individuals with dementia may be eligible for financial help as well as healthcare coverage through these programs.

4. Support groups: Contact groups that specialize in dementia care. They frequently offer resources, instructional materials, and guidance in resolving legal and financial difficulties.

5. Investigate local community services that provide assistance to people with dementia and their families. Legal clinics, financial counseling, and caregiver support groups are examples of such services.

In conclusion, legal and financial considerations are critical in the dementia journey. Individuals and their families can negotiate this challenging terrain with better confidence and preparedness by planning for the future, resolving challenges, and gaining access to resources.

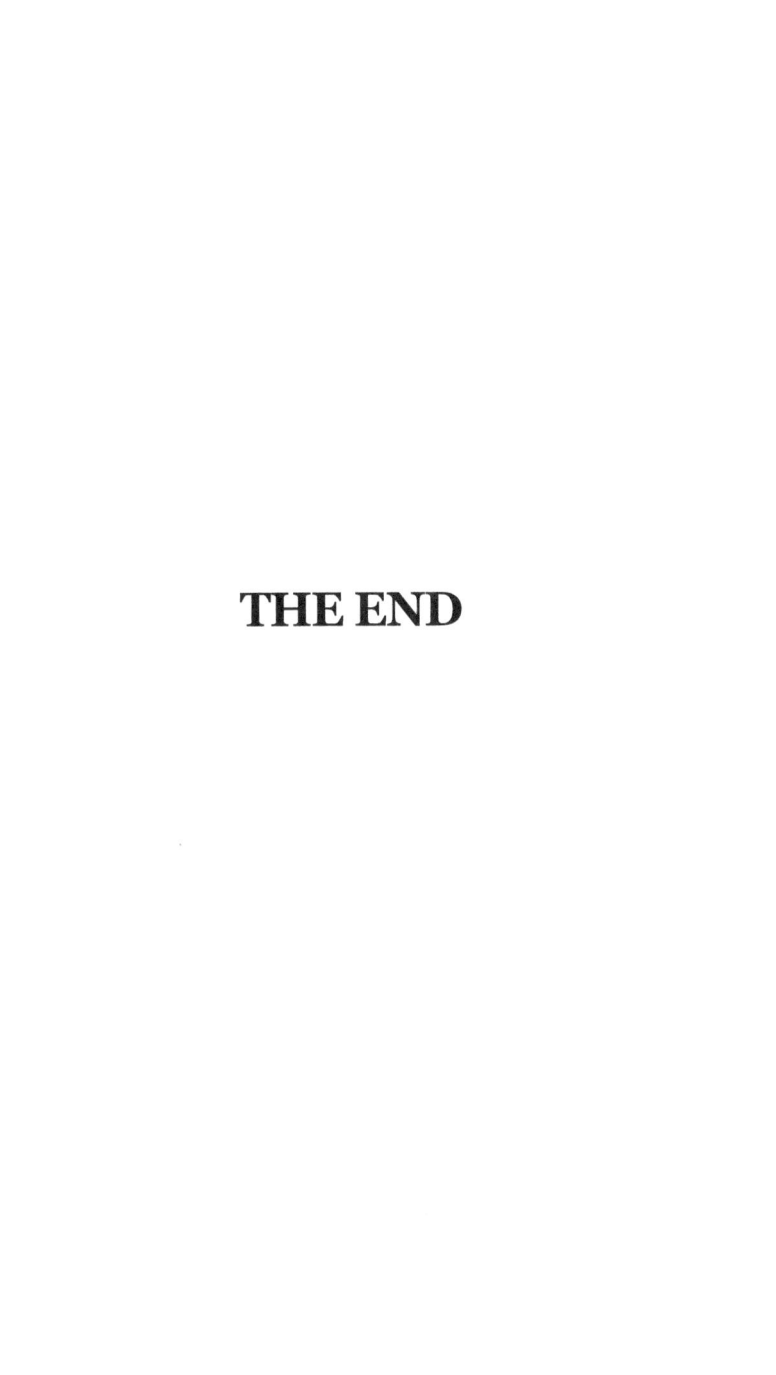

THE END